THE HOSPICE Q & A BOOK

ADVOCATING FOR YOUR LOVED ONES

JoAnn Barmettler

THE HOSPICE Q & A BOOK
Advocating For Your Loved Ones
By JoAnn Barmettler

Copyright © 2025

All rights reserved.

Printed in the United States of America

Editing and Formatting
Cover Design by Teagarden Designs
The Hospice Q&A Book
Advocating For Your Loved Ones

Copyright @ 2025 JoAnn Barmettler
Name: JoAnn Barmettler, author
Title: The Hospice Q&A Book
Website: https://joannbarmettler.com/

ISBN:
978-1-80558-538-1 = Ebook
978-1-80558-539-8 = Pkaperback
978-1-80558-540-4 = Hardcover

What Others Are Saying About JoAnn Barmettler

"This book is the secret blueprint that every person involved in a hospice event can use to get closer to understanding just how hospice works. JoAnn Barmettler has put together a unique collection of life lessons and personal success stories to capture one's heart and soul. Her book is incredibly noteworthy, valuable, and inspiring to help you and your loved ones achieve a wonderful and fulfilling end-of-life hospice experience. "The Hospice Q & A Book" is truly magical! Well done!"

—**John Formica,** The "Ex-Disney Guy"
America's Customer Experience Speaker
and Coach at www.JohnFornica.com

"JoAnn Barmettler's leadership skills, honed through her military service and nursing career, enable her to effectively lead and advocate for individuals and families in healthcare and hospice settings. This book is a must-read!"

—**Jill Lublin,** 4X Best Selling Author,
International Speaker,
Master Publicity Strategist

"JoAnn Barmettler is an expert practitioner in the art and science of medicine. Her book has helped guide my family through the difficult process of deciding to seek hospice care and what to expect along the journey. I highly recommend this book for patients, families along with clinicians involved in compassionate end of life care."

—**Colonel John F. Detro,** United States
Special Operations Command Surgeon

"If you're searching for a healthcare advocate and leader who will go above and beyond to ensure the best possible care for your loved ones, look no further than JoAnn Barmettler."

—**Megan Unsworth,** Co-founder of LifeonFire.com
Queen of Coaching

"With a career spanning three decades in the healthcare industry, JoAnn Barmettler has cemented her reputation as a formidable authority and captivating speaker on health and wellness issues. As someone who has had the privilege of experiencing her presentations firsthand, I can attest to her prowess and engagement as a speaker. I therefore enthusiastically endorse her as an excellent choice for any event or forum seeking an impactful and informative keynote. JoAnn's depth and breadth of knowledge in the healthcare industry is truly unrivaled. Yet, what sets her apart is her rare ability to distill complex medical concepts into digestible information that resonates with audiences of all backgrounds. Her unique blend of expertise and relatability ensures that everyone, regardless of their level of medical understanding, leaves her sessions enlightened and empowered."

—**Twanda "Tia" Young,** Brigadier General (Retired)

EDUCATE OTHERS

"SHARE THIS BOOK"

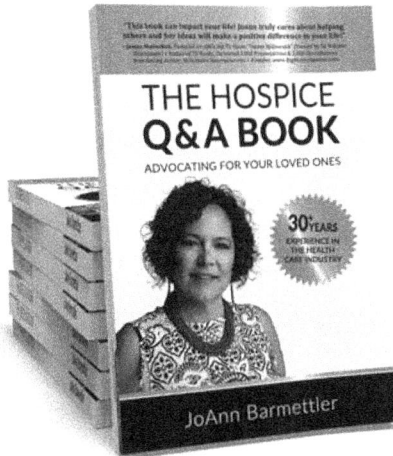

RETAIL $19.97

SPECIAL QUANTITY DISCOUNTS

5-20 Books	$17.97
21-99 Books	$15.97
100-499 Books	$13.97
500-999 Books	$11.97
1000+ Books	$9.97

TO PLACE AND ORDER CONTACT:

jlbarmettler@gmail.com

www.joannbarmettler.com

THE IDEA PROFESSIONAL SPEAKER FOR YOUR NEXT EVENT!

Any organization that wants to develop their people to have invaluable perspectives about hospice, needs to hire JoAnn for a keynote and/or workshop training!

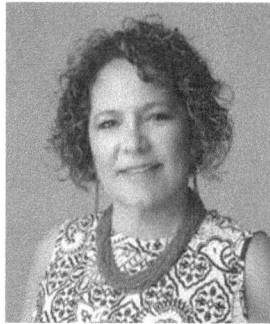

TO CONTACT OR BOOK JOANN TO SPEAK:

jlbarmettler@gmail.com

www.joannbarmettler.com

I dedicate this book to many loved ones that have passed in hospice care. Including my father Guy, age 57; my father-in-law Gerald, age 59; my mother Sue, age 72; my brother Otis, age 50; and my mother-in-law Shirley, age 82. Plus, the many other loved ones that passed in hospice care. I miss them all.

I thank everybody who trusted me enough to call me and allow me to help them with their loved ones who needed hospice care.

I pray for each of you as you read this book. May you be empowered, blessed, and strengthened through the process for your loved one.

Most lovingly, I thank my amazing husband, Tim Barmettler. You have been a blessing to many families and me. You did things to help them when they were in need. When I had families call me late at night, and it wasn't my turn to be on call, you always told me to go because they trusted me and needed me.

Thank you for having a giving and kind heart.

Tim, you are a true blessing!

FOREWARD

You may remember me from being featured on the hit ABC TV show, "Secret Millionaire." If you do not know of the show, here is the basic premise from show promotions: "What happens when business motivational speaker and self-made millionaire James Malinchak is picked up by an ABC television crew, placed on an airplane with no money, credit cards, cell phone, laptop or watch, and is whisked off to an impoverished neighborhood, where he had to survive on $44.66 cents for a week?

The show features Malinchak leaving his current lifestyle in search of real-life heroes who are making a difference in their local community. He ultimately reveals himself as a millionaire and rewards them with a portion of his own money to further their cause by gifting them with checks of his own money totaling over $100,000. If you watched ABC's 'Secret Millionaire' you know that James is no ordinary entrepreneur. He is a self-made millionaire with a strong passion for giving back and serving others."

Amazingly, over 50 MIILLION+ people watched the show! Whether I am speaking at a conference, walking through an airport, consulting for an entrepreneur or just hanging out at a coffee shop, I always seem to get asked the same question. "What was it like being on Secret Millionaire when you had to live undercover in an impoverished neighborhood and how did it affect you?"

My answer is always the same.

The greatest gift you can have is when you simply give, in order to help and serve others. There is no better feeling than when you know you have made a positive difference in the lives of others.

And that is exactly what JoAnn, and her information can do for you! JoAnn will inspire you through sharing her wisdom and personal experiences.

JoAnn is a coach, author, speaker, and seminar leader who truly cares about making a positive difference in the lives of others.

In this book you will be inspired by JoAnn's genuine, caring nature for making a difference. And her strategies can help you to improve all areas of your life.

Some strategies may comfort you while others may challenge your old paradigm. One thing is for certain. JoAnn and her strategies will stamp your spirit with an abundance of love, hope and encouragement so you can reach new levels of courage, fulfillment, and personal happiness.

It is my sincere honor to introduce to you JoAnn and her brilliant book!

—**James Malinchak,** Featured on ABCs Hit TV Show, "Secret
Millionaire" (Viewed by 50 Million+ Worldwide)
Authored 25 Books, Delivered 3,000 Presentations
& 2,000 Consultations
Best-Selling Author, Millionaire Success Secrets
Founder, www.BigMoneySpeaker.com

CONTENTS

INTRODUCTION

Are you aware that each year, approximately three million people seek hospice services? That's roughly equivalent to 8,219 individuals per day.

I am composing this book based on my extensive involvement with hospice care, during which I have witnessed numerous remarkable experiences as well as a few less-than-ideal ones. Given these experiences, my aim is to prevent anyone from having a negative encounter with hospice. If you find yourself needing hospice care for a loved one, my hope is that this book equips you with the knowledge and resources to ensure the best possible experience, one that offers your loved one the peace and comfort they deserve as they depart this world.

My name is JoAnn, and I have dedicated over 15 years to serving as a hospice nurse, in addition to advocating for hospice for more than 25 years. Over the years, I've worn multiple hats in the context of hospice care: I've been the nurse, the daughter, the sister, the niece, and the friend to those who have embarked on their hospice journey.

Interestingly, once people discover that I am a hospice nurse, they often open-up about their own experiences with hospice, both positive and negative. I frequently receive inquiries from friends, acquaintances, and even strangers seeking advice on how to navigate hospice care for their loved ones. Many of these individuals' express feelings of confusion or uncertainty about the process, prompting me to extend my guidance and support whenever it is needed.

I vividly recall an incident at an Army conference where I overheard a soldier discussing hospice. He seemed almost incredulous, and I couldn't help but interject. I introduced myself as a hospice nurse and offered my assistance, sensing that he might be in need. He explained that the doctor had recently recommended hospice for their mother and asked if I would be willing to speak with his sister, who was the power of attorney for their mother.

As I elucidated the concept of hospice care to her, I assured her that I could assist her throughout the process and shared my contact information. We conducted interviews with various hospice companies over the phone until we identified the one that best suited their mother's needs. I provided guidance on what questions to ask, what to anticipate, and how to make the most of their mother's remaining days. This guidance not only benefitted their mother but also brought solace to the entire family.

The soldier frequently texted me during this process, expressing gratitude for the help they had received. They felt that their experience was significantly more positive than they had initially anticipated. Their mother's final days were characterized by laughter, joy, and rekindled relationships with family members who had been distant. She experienced peace and was free from pain—precisely how it should be.

For those currently facing the challenge of hospice care for a loved one, my aspiration is that your experience surpasses your expectations, much like the gentleman soldier described in his mother's case. I want you to feel empowered and self-assured after perusing this book. You will gain a comprehensive understanding of what to anticipate and the questions to pose.

I pledge to provide you with the information and tools necessary to navigate this demanding process successfully. Hospice care is emotionally charged when a loved one is involved, and the inability to control the situation can lead to frustration. Regardless of where you stand in this process or if you're assisting a friend, I will equip you with the resources required to ensure a smooth transition for your loved one.

CHAPTER 1

WHAT IS HOSPICE?

WHAT IS HOSPICE?

Hospice is dedicated to delivering care that emphasizes comfort, dignity, and emotional support for both the patient and their family. The paramount objective is to enhance the quality of life. Rather than pursuing a cure, hospice focuses on symptom management and pain relief. Choosing hospice is not a surrender; it signifies a commitment to prioritizing comfort and an improved quality of life for as long as possible. The approach is customized to meet the individual needs of each client, with an interdisciplinary team overseeing pain management, symptom control, and tailored care plans.

Hospice offers additional support during the end of life, and it grants patients the option to remain in their preferred setting, often their own homes. For those who choose to stay home, provided it is safe, they can do so in the familiar and comforting environment of their residence. Necessary items for comfort, such as walkers, wheelchairs, hospital beds, and medications, are brought to the patient's home by the hospice team.

In cases requiring hospitalization, hospital staff will administer care, comfort medications, and any other necessary support. Hospice services can be provided in various settings, including the patient's home, assisted living facilities, nursing homes, hospitals, or hospice houses. Many individuals express a wish to spend their final moments in the comfort of their own homes, and whenever feasible, hospice strives to fulfill this preference.

Furthermore, hospice offers a wide array of resources, not only for the patient but also for their family, throughout the journey of end-of-life care.

"To know even one life has breathed easier because you have lived, that is to have succeeded."

~ Ralph Waldo Emmerson ~

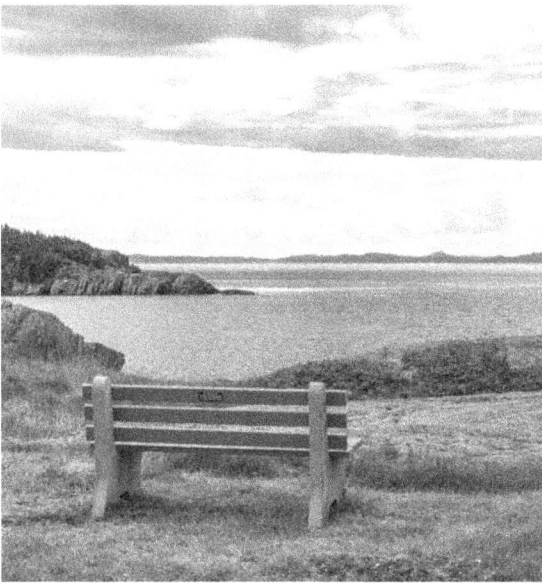

NOTES

CHAPTER 2

WHAT DO YOU GET WHEN YOU HAVE HOSPICE?

WHAT DO YOU GET WHEN YOU HAVE HOSPICE?

You will have access to a comprehensive team of professionals, including a nurse's aide, nurse, social worker, and chaplain, as well as a medical director who can collaborate with your primary physician or take the lead in addressing End-of-life symptoms to ensure comfort. These symptoms may encompass pain, breathing difficulties, personal grief, wounds, and anxiety. The team is equipped to address any physical, emotional, or spiritual needs that may arise, often offering the invaluable presence of a volunteer for added comfort and companionship.

Additionally, the team provides essential medications and medical equipment, such as briefs, wipes, wheelchairs, hospital beds, and bedside commodes, among others, to enhance your loved one's comfort. Hospice covers the cost of medications related to the diagnosed condition for which your loved one has been admitted.

Typically, the nurse's aide will visit twice a week to provide bathing and any assistance needed to enhance comfort. The nurse's frequency of visits varies depending on symptoms and the severity of the disease, typically ranging from two to three times a week for home patients and two times a week for nursing home patients. However, it's important to note that each hospice company may have different visitation schedules, so it's advisable to inquire for specific details. As symptoms or conditions change, additional visits are usually scheduled.

The social worker conducts an initial assessment to identify any additional needs or resources that should be included in the care plan. Subsequently, they make follow-up visits one to two times a month, depending on the ongoing requirements for extra support.

The chaplain is available at the patient's request, and it is recommended that they be included in the care plan regardless of religious beliefs. Their role is primarily to listen and provide guidance, assisting patients with end-of-life beliefs, thoughts, and struggles without attempting to alter their beliefs. The chaplain helps prepare the patient for the next phase of their journey. In situations where patients initially decline a chaplain visit, it's often suggested that they allow at least one visit. Most of the time, patients find comfort in sharing with the chaplain, even more so than with the nurse or aide.

For instance, a client's experience illustrates the significance of chaplaincy involvement. Despite initially desiring only her pastor's presence, the client met with the chaplain and engaged in a nearly two-hour conversation, sharing vital information that had not been disclosed to anyone else. This interaction helped her address unresolved issues and allowed the hospice team to better manage her pain.

The medical director collaborates closely with the nurse to guide medical management, ensuring the best possible care for the patient. They are readily available for consultation, including new orders and symptom management as needed.

The patient has the option to retain their personal physician if the physician is willing to collaborate with the nursing team to oversee the patient's care. In many cases, personal physicians lack expertise in hospice medications, and their suitability may not always be optimal. It is advisable to discuss with the patient's physician whether they are willing and experienced in hospice medications and whether they can be reached for consultation at any time, day, or night.

Hospice does not offer round-the-clock in-home care but does ensure 24-hour accessibility to the nurse and any other necessary personnel involved in the patient's care.

"I wonder if my first breath was as soul stirring to my mother as her last breath was to me?"

~ Lisa Goich Andreadis ~

NOTES

CHAPTER 3

WHAT ARE THE 8 MYTHS ABOUT HOSPICE?

WHAT ARE THE 8 MYTHS ABOUT HOSPICE?

There are misconceptions circulating about hospice services, including false beliefs that using hospice means foregoing access to food, water, medications, or antibiotics. These misconceptions are often referred to as myths because they are not accurate. I've encountered a variety of such unfounded beliefs from people.

1 THEY CANNOT GO INTO HOSPICE CARE BECAUSE THEY WON'T GIVE THEM ANY WATER OR FOOD AND THAT'S A CRUEL WAY TO DIE.

Fact: When under hospice care, individuals are permitted to eat and drink if they are physically capable, and their dietary preferences are respected. In the context of a progressive disease, the body's natural processes change, and it no longer experiences hunger or thirst in the same way as before. Patients can continue to enjoy their preferred foods and drinks until the very end of life.

It's important to emphasize caution regarding the last statement. It's not uncommon for families to be unaware of the physiological changes occurring in their loved one's body during this phase. It is never advisable to pressure or force a loved one to consume food when they do not wish to.

Illustration: My mother-in-law had diabetes, which necessitated regular blood sugar monitoring before meals. When she transitioned into hospice care, I broached the topic of whether she wished to continue monitoring her blood sugar levels. I made it clear that the decision was entirely up to her, and she was not obliged to do so. After we explained the physiological changes occurring in her body, she chose not to continue monitoring. Initially, there were a few family members who wanted to persist with blood sugar checks until we clarified that this was her personal decision, rooted in the understanding of the physiological process.

My mother-in-law felt that if her life was drawing to a close, there was no need to restrict her diet. She expressed a desire to savor some sweet treats, and we honored her choice. She enjoyed a variety of delicious foods until her appetite waned, and the disease process eventually ran its course.

2 THEY WILL JUST TRY TO KILL YOU OFF WITH MORPHINE, WHICH IS HOW THEY DIE.

Fact: Administering an overdose of morphine is a challenging and uncommon way for individuals to pass away. When someone is in hospice care, their primary condition is what leads to the decline in their health, not the appropriate management of pain. It's crucial to emphasize that effectively addressing pain at the end of life does not hasten a person's death. Instead, the disease process progresses, leading to the gradual failure of bodily organs. At this stage, the body loses its ability to maintain homeostasis.

3 I WILL HAVE TO LEAVE MY OWN HOME AND BECOME AN IN-PATIENT SOMEWHERE.

Fact: Hospice is not a physical location; it represents a care philosophy. Hospice care is provided wherever the patient considers home, whether it's their own residence, an assisted living facility, a nursing home, an inpatient hospice facility, or a hospital.

You have the flexibility to choose where you receive hospice care based on your preferences and safety considerations. If it's safe for you to stay at home, hospice services can be provided there. In some areas, you may find facilities known as "Hospice Houses" or similar names, designed to accommodate patients who require hospice care and cannot stay at home for various reasons.

These facilities are staffed by professionals trained in hospice care, just like the teams from hospice companies. The hospice company will continue to provide care and support when you or your loved one is in a hospice house. It's important to inquire about any daily room charges associated with a "Hospice House" before deciding.

4 HOSPICE CARE IS EXPENSIVE.

Fact: Hospice care is typically covered by Medicare, Medicaid, and most insurance plans. While some insurance companies may require a co-payment for hospice services, many hospices also handle "pro-bono" cases. In cases where a patient lacks Medicare, Medicaid, or insurance coverage, a hospice company may still admit them for care, even if they will not receive reimbursement for the provided services and expenses.

5 HOSPICE IS JUST FOR PEOPLE WITH CANCER DIAGNOSIS.

Fact: Hospice care is available to individuals of all age groups who are dealing with a life-limiting illness. In my experience, I have provided care to hospice patients for periods exceeding three years. This extended duration is due to the presence of a debilitating disease process that did not offer the prospect of improvement.

6 IF IT'S TIME FOR HOSPICE, MY DOCTOR WILL TELL ME ABOUT IT AND RECOMMEND IT.

Fact: It's important to initiate a conversation about hospice care with your doctor as early as possible. Regrettably, some doctors may never broach the subject of hospice with their patients. Many physicians harbor concerns that they are letting their patients down by introducing the topic of hospice. I've had numerous physician friends express this sentiment to me until I provided them with information about hospice and its processes.

Choosing to have a conversation about "hospice" does not signify a failure on the part of the doctor. Rather, it demonstrates their commitment to enhancing their patients' quality of life, particularly when the disease has advanced beyond the possibility of a cure or recovery. (Please refer to Otis' story in the "Hospice Stories" section for further insight.)

7 HOSPICE MEANS PATIENTS MUST DIE WITHIN SIX MONTHS.

Fact: Hospice care is typically available to individuals with a prognosis of six months or less to live, although some patients exceed this timeframe significantly. Patients continue to receive hospice services as long as they remain suitable for hospice care, which means their condition is deteriorating, and a cure for their disease process is unlikely. Indicators of appropriateness for hospice may include weight loss, recurrent infections, frequent hospitalizations, or falls, among other symptoms that suggest the progression of the disease.

For instance, my uncle, who has Chronic Obstructive Pulmonary Disease (COPD) and a history of bladder cancer, began experiencing recurrent infections, frequent hospitalizations, and falls. When we approached his primary care doctor about hospice, the response was initially negative. However, after consulting with a cardiologist who concurred that my uncle met the criteria for hospice, an order was issued for a hospice evaluation, resulting in his admission on the same day. At the time of writing, he has been receiving hospice care for a month. While we cannot predict how much longer he will live, the management of his symptoms at home has provided both him and his family with peace. This experience has underscored the importance of advocating for him and his family.

In many cases, individuals have conditions that will not improve, such as dementia, and they qualify for hospice services. Some patients with dementia have received hospice care for one to two years, with the duration dependent on how the disease has affected their body. Hospice admission is based on appropriateness rather than an attempt to predict a specific timeframe for the end of life.

Illustration: I once cared for a hospice patient afflicted with congestive heart failure. She had endured multiple hospital admissions, prompting her doctor, who happened to be a friend of mine, to reach out and inquire if there was anything hospice could do to assist her. After assessment, she met the criteria for hospice care and was admitted, allowing us to manage her disease process within the comforts of her home.

As a nurse, I had the ability to discern shifts in her condition indicating a deterioration of symptoms. This insight enabled me to adapt medication regimens to avert emergency room visits or hospital stays. This proactive approach involved close coordination with the hospice medical director. Above all, we had the privilege of honoring her heartfelt wish to pass away at home, surrounded by the presence of her cherished loved ones.

8 ONCE YOU ARE ADMITTED TO THE HOSPICE YOU MUST STAY IN HOSPICE CARE.

Fact: Hospice patients maintain the right to opt for a return to conventional medical care at any point. Regardless of the reason or timing, if a patient decides to shift their focus back to treatments aimed at curing their illness or addressing their disease, they have the autonomy to do so. If a previously discharged patient later wishes to re-enter hospice care, most insurance providers typically permit re-admission.

For instance, there was an 85-year-old lady under hospice care due to a decline in her overall well-being. Following medication adjustments, her condition markedly improved, leading to her transition out of hospice care.

It is crucial to prioritize accurate information to make informed decisions concerning your loved ones or offer support to friends, thereby dispelling the misconceptions that circulate about hospice care. Often, these myths persist because individuals simply hear rumors without verifying the facts. Unfortunately, some individuals have endured unnecessary suffering because their family members or friends failed to research or seek the truth about hospice care. It's worth noting that doctors, like all of us, are human and may not possess all-encompassing knowledge.

NOTES

_____
_____
_____
_____
_____
_____
_____
_____
_____
_____
_____
_____
_____
_____
_____
_____

CHAPTER 4

WHAT ARE THE SIX BENEFITS OF HOSPICE?

WHAT ARE THE SIX BENEFITS OF HOSPICE?

1 HOSPICE RESPECTS INDIVIDUAL GOALS AND PRIORITIES.

Many individuals often overlook the advantages of hospice care, such as the emphasis on ensuring the comfort of their loved ones and effectively addressing and managing their symptoms. It's important to acknowledge that, at times, finding the right approach may involve a degree of trial and error. I have encountered challenging cases involving patients with rare diseases, for whom effectively managing their pain posed a considerable challenge. However, we remained steadfast in our commitment, diligently working to alleviate their pain, and affording both the patients and their loved ones the opportunity for meaningful and quality conversations.

2 HOSPICE SUPPORTS FAMILY AND CAREGIVERS.

The support provided extends beyond the patient to encompass the family as well. It is crucial to aid family members in comprehending the significance of hospice care. Unfortunately, many individuals hold a negative perception of hospice, often stemming from hearing unfavorable stories or experiences from friends or loved ones. In some cases, a doctor may have delayed in making a hospice referral, or the option of hospice care may not have been adequately communicated to them, resulting in their loved one passing away either at home or in the hospital without the comfort of being surrounded by loved ones.

3 HOSPICE CARE MAINTAINS AND PROMOTES DIGNITY, AND HONORS PATIENT WISHES.

We had a patient who lacked immediate family, but he had legal representation through the court in the form of power of attorney. His expressed desire was to pass away in the comfort of his own home, a wish we were determined to fulfill. To make this happen, we coordinated resources and arrangements with his court-appointed power of attorney. While I can't guarantee this outcome in every case, I can confidently say that we come very close to making it happen as often as possible.

4 HOSPICE LESSENS THE FINANCIAL BURDEN.

Hospice provides a comprehensive array of resources readily available for your loved one's care, addressing their needs without incurring additional expenses for you.

5 HOSPICE INCLUDES A TEAM OF SPECIALISTS.

Having specialists involved in our loved ones' care is crucial, especially if we are not in the healthcare field. However, even for those in healthcare, the specialized knowledge and expertise of hospice may be unfamiliar or essential.

6 HOSPICE OFFERS A FAMILIAR ENVIRONMENT.

As a hospice nurse, my primary goal is to do my utmost to fulfill my patients' wishes, ensuring that the situation is safe and supported with the necessary resources. There are instances when a patient is better cared for in a hospice house, especially if their home environment poses safety concerns.

I recall a poignant experience with a World War II Veteran who was resolute about remaining in his home, and rightfully so. One night, his daughter urgently called me for a visit as he was becoming increasingly restless. Upon arriving at his bedside, he requested that his family leave the room. What followed was a heartfelt confession of wartime experiences and actions that had burdened him for decades.

Recognizing the need for him to discuss these long-held secrets, I explained to his family that he required a safe space to open-up about his wartime past. It was common for individuals facing the end of life to withhold such confessions, not because they were sins, but because they carried the weight of those memories for so long and felt the need to unburden themselves.

This Veteran had, in fact, protected himself during a harrowing period in history. As a fellow Veteran, we engaged in extensive conversations about his experiences. He cried and sobbed, releasing the emotional weight he had carried for years. I listened, offered prayers, and, by the end of our visit, he expressed relief.

Before reuniting him with his family, he grasped my hand and conveyed his gratitude for enabling him to remain in his home and find peace in his final moments. It was remarkable how he appeared decades younger, radiating a newfound sense of peace. His family also noticed the transformation, and they cherished their last few days together, marked by laughter, tears, and shared memories.

The patient passed away several days later, but his family recounted the profound impact of those final moments. They spoke of how they laughed, cried, and reminisced together, describing it as an incredible experience. They believed their father had transformed into a different person after our visit, where he had openly sobbed and made his long-awaited confession. I explained that he had unburdened himself of a heavy weight, finally feeling relieved and free to be himself.

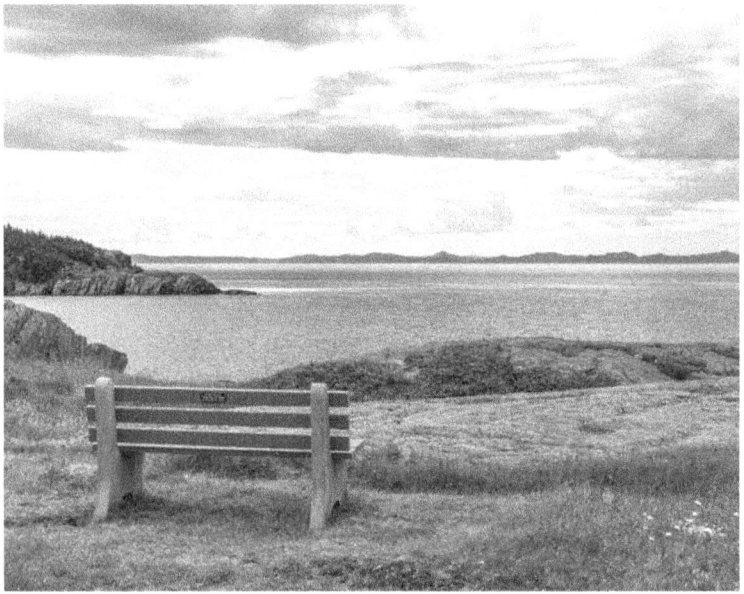

"At the end of life what really matters is not what we bought, but what we built, not what we got but what we shared; not our competence, but our character; and not our success but our significance. Live a life that matters. Live a life of love."

~Unknown~

NOTES

CHAPTER 5

WHERE DO I BEGIN IF I THINK MY LOVED ONE NEEDS HOSPICE?

WHERE DO I BEGIN IF I THINK MY LOVED ONE NEEDS HOSPICE?

Consult with your Doctor: If your doctor is receptive, you can request them to provide a referral to your chosen hospice service. The referral should specify that you want the hospice company to evaluate and admit your loved one if deemed appropriate.

Select a Suitable Hospice Company: Once you've made your choice, ask your doctor's office to fax the order to the selected hospice company, including the most recent medical history, physical examination records, current medication list, and any details about recent surgeries, treatments, or hospitalizations. This information will help the hospice team gain a comprehensive understanding of your loved one's condition.

Hospice Assessment: The hospice company will thoroughly review all the provided information and then contact you to arrange an assessment of your loved one.

Admission Process: After the assessment, if your loved one qualifies for hospice care, the hospice company will guide you through the remaining admission and care processes.

When Your Doctor Disagrees: If your doctor is unwilling to consider hospice care, contact a hospice company of your choice and explain your situation. You can inquire about other doctors within the hospice network who may be willing to discuss the situation with you. It's essential to prioritize the well-being of the patient, and if the current doctor is not open to the idea of hospice, exploring other options is necessary.

It's worth noting that I have personal experience in both facilitating hospice care and being a family member receiving hospice support. This dual perspective has equipped me to provide insights into how the process should ideally function.

A crucial starting point is asking questions. By maintaining a curious attitude and seeking answers to your inquiries, you demonstrate your commitment to ensuring the best care for your loved one. When I began this journey, the internet was relatively new and not as efficient for obtaining quick information. Nowadays, with the internet readily available, it's much easier to access accurate information swiftly.

While medical personnel might not always appreciate extensive questioning, it's important to remember that asking questions does not signify distrust or questioning their expertise. Rather, it demonstrates your dedication to becoming an informed advocate. I, as a nurse, went through nursing school and understood the significance of asking questions when I encountered something I didn't fully grasp. This was essential for both my future patients and me.

In your role, as you navigate the hospice process, asking questions is vital to understanding what to expect and making informed decisions, whether it involves surgery, chemotherapy, new medications, or opting for hospice care. Asking questions is your pathway to obtaining the answers you need to determine the best course of action for your loved one's well-being.

"Hospice is such a
tremendous thing.
Patients seem to reach
an inner peace."

~ Harmon Killebrew ~

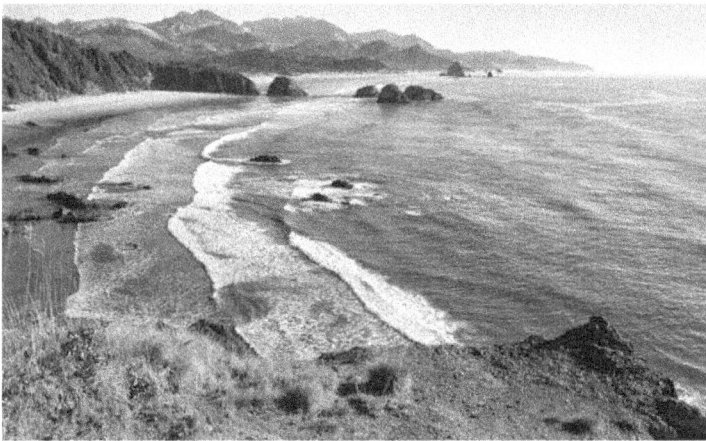

NOTES

CHAPTER 6

WHAT QUESTIONS DO I ASK WHEN INTERVIEWING HOSPICE COMPANIES?

WHEN INTERVIEWING HOSPICE COMPANIES?

When most doctors recommend a hospice, they usually recommend the hospice company they are most familiar with. That does not mean that will be the right hospice company for you and your loved one. You have the right to interview different hospice companies. A list can be provided for you, or you can google the hospice companies in your area.

Regardless, interview different companies. I have worked for a couple different hospice companies, and I prefer one over the other, but overall, I was grateful they didn't put time restraints or resource constraints on us with our patients.

Questions To Ask the Hospice Company

1. What do you provide for my loved one on hospice care?

2. How often do the following team members' visits take place? Nurse, aide, social worker, pastor, and volunteer?

3. What if my family needs some added resources?

4. If I need something, such as a hospital bed or another medication needed to manage symptoms for my loved one, how soon can I expect somebody to come and help with the situation?

5. How long has your medical director been on board with hospice or how much hospice experience do they have?

6. What if I am unhappy with a team member or the personality does not work well with my family or loved one?

7. When needing resources who decides whether we can get what is needed?

8. Is your company run by a corporation that makes all the decisions or is your company allowed to make decisions at this level?

9. Once we choose to sign up for the hospice care, how long does it take to get the equipment we need?

10. Are there only certain medications you use? Such as if we request a certain pain medication that you don't normally use, can we get it regardless of cost?

11. *Please read Ron's story under Hospice Stories.

12. When calling the hospice company for a nursing issue what is the normal response time? See Ron's story in the back of the book.

13. What is the mission of your hospice company?

14. How long has this company been around?

15. Do you have a high turnover of your staff?

NOTES

CHAPTER 7

WHAT TO DO WHEN FAMILY MEMBERS ARE RESISTANT TO HOSPICE?

WHAT TO DO WHEN FAMILY MEMBERS ARE RESISTANT TO HOSPICE?

Many individuals exhibit resistance towards hospice, often stemming from negative past experiences, hearsay from friends, or simply a lack of understanding about what hospice entails. In such situations, it's crucial to uncover the root of this resistance. I recall a meeting with a family regarding hospice care for their mother. Among the ten children, the decision-makers were in favor of hospice, while others were not. Recognizing the importance of unanimous agreement, I suggested gathering all the siblings for a discussion.

Upon their arrival, I personally greeted each family member and initiated the conversation by asking, "What is causing your hesitation towards hospice?" I encouraged them to be candid and open about their concerns. Addressing each objection, I provided education, support, and listened with empathy and compassion.

To illustrate the significance of hospice, I shared my personal story about my father's experience. Subsequently, I asked each sibling to jot down what they believed their mother would want on a piece of paper. One son grew upset and left the room, while others murmured disapproval about his behavior. I took the opportunity to have a one-on-one conversation with him.

Even though he wasn't the power of attorney, I inquired about his life and upbringing. He confided that he felt responsible for his mother's situation and believed he had let her down in some way. Our conversation focused on addressing these feelings, and I encouraged him to communicate with his mother, expressing his love and concerns, emphasizing that he may not have many more chances.

In essence, his resistance was rooted in the fear of letting go and the misconception that he had caused his mother's situation. After our discussion, filled with understanding, education, and empathy, he became supportive of the hospice decision. When he shared this change of heart with his siblings, they were visibly surprised. The oldest sister, one of the powers of attorney, inquired about what I had said to change his mind. I emphasized that it wasn't just my words but the act of listening and validating his feelings and concerns.

Every individual processes these decisions differently, and family dynamics, upbringing, personal favorites, and the presence or absence of parents can all contribute to these emotions. The decision to admit a loved one to hospice often involves a complex interplay of emotions, resembling a circus with multiple acts, each representing different emotions, unfolding simultaneously.

Throughout my work in hospice, I learned to appreciate the unique dynamics of each family and the emotional complexity involved in these decisions. My role involved listening with empathy and validating feelings, acknowledging that everyone has the right to their emotions and opinions, regardless of their accuracy. This is where the value of having a hospice team comes into play. Hospice professionals excel at working with families, including hesitant members, by providing education and validating their emotions.

In situations where a family member remains unconvinced, hospice can step in to facilitate a conversation or involve someone they respect and trust who possesses knowledge about hospice care.

"Endings matter, not just for the person but, perhaps even more, for the ones left behind."

~ Atul Gawande ~

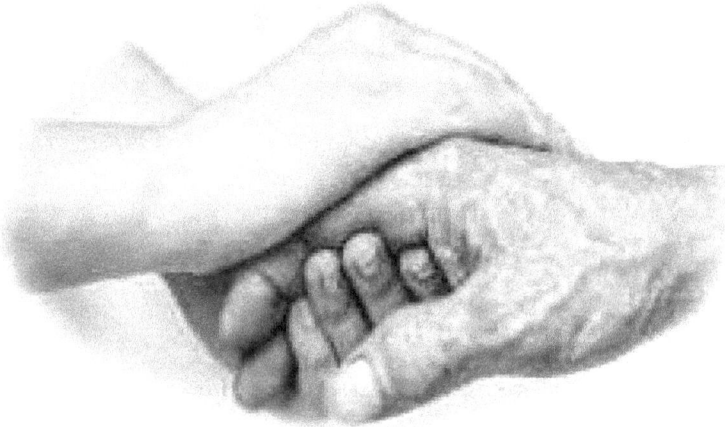

NOTES

CHAPTER 8

WHAT DO YOU SAY WHEN THE END NEARS?

WHAT DO YOU SAY WHEN THE END NEARS?

Families often wonder what to say when their loved ones are on hospice care, assuming that unresponsive patients cannot hear them. However, this is not the case, as they can still hear everything happening around them. Allow me to share the heartwarming story of Maria, one of my favorite patients, to illustrate the power of communication during this time.

Maria, a lovely 90-year-old woman under hospice care, had been unconscious for about three days, indicating that the end was approaching. Her granddaughter was preparing for her wedding, and it was Maria's heartfelt wish to attend. I advised her granddaughter to start sharing every detail of her wedding with her grandmother. She did so for approximately 30-40 minutes, describing the wedding in detail.

Later, Maria's daughter requested that we pray together, and we did. Surprisingly, as I was praying, Maria suddenly woke up and exclaimed, "I can hear everything you are saying; I am right here. Now, I want to hear more about the wedding." She remained awake for the next three hours, engaging in a clear and lively conversation with her granddaughter and daughter about the upcoming wedding. Afterward, she returned to an unconscious state and passed away the following day.

While not everyone gets such a remarkable opportunity, the significance lies in the content of your conversations with your loved ones, whether they are conscious or not. I have observed many instances where restless patients were calmed when their families began discussing memories.

Here are some strategies for meaningful communication during this time:

- **Use "I remember when" statements:** Recall special moments and share stories, such as humorous anecdotes or cherished memories. For example, "I remember when Dad did this, and we laughed for hours."

- **Reminisce about enjoyable activities:** Reflect on fun activities or experiences you shared together. Encourage reminiscing by asking, "Do you remember when we did this or that?"

- **Express love and appreciation:** Tell your loved one what you love most about them and express your feelings from the heart.

- **Offer reassurance:** Let your loved one know that you will be okay when they pass, providing them with peace of mind. Assure them that you will carry on their legacy by maintaining certain traditions or cherished aspects of their life.

- **Play their favorite music:** If your loved one enjoys music, play their favorite songs softly in the background. Music can be soothing and comforting.

Laughter is a wonderful way to lift spirits, and the laughter of children and grandchildren can be especially uplifting. While some may be concerned about having children around, their presence can bring peace to restless loved ones. Children's innocent and joyful chatter often has a calming effect.

I recall a situation when my mother was in her final hours. She was growing restless, and I realized that there were a few grandchildren she hadn't seen or heard from in a while. I called them and asked them to visit as soon as possible, sensing that their voices would bring comfort to her.

When they arrived, I coached each grandchild on what to say. They shared stories about school, talked about their Christmas break, and mentioned funny memories with their grandmother. They also expressed what they loved most about her and offered kisses or held her hand while speaking to her. These heartfelt interactions had a remarkable impact, as my mother visibly relaxed, smiled, and even seemed to respond.

Make the most of your remaining moments together. This is not the time for family disagreements or conflicts. Instead, cherish these precious moments, ensuring that your loved one's last experiences are filled with joy and peace. Let the last things they hear bring them comfort and serenity.

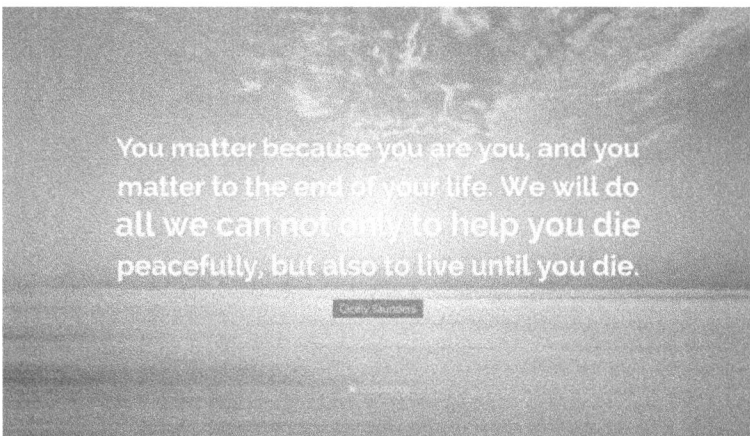

You matter because you are you, and you matter to the end of your life. We will do all we can not only to help you die peacefully, but also to live until you die.

Cicely Saunders

NOTES

CHAPTER 9

WHAT IF MY LOVED ONE IMPROVES WITH HOSPICE?

WHAT IF MY LOVED ONE IMPROVES WITH HOSPICE?

This scenario is not uncommon, and I've had the privilege of witnessing many older patients "graduate" from hospice care. One memorable case involved a patient we'll call Jane, who was initially admitted to hospice with the diagnosis of "failure to thrive." Jane's condition was deteriorating rapidly, and it appeared that she might have been overmedicated. She was hardly eating, barely responsive to stimuli, and seemed to be in a steep decline.

After consulting with the family, we made the decision to gradually reduce Jane's medications. As we began this process, we started to notice remarkable improvements in her alertness, appetite, and overall awareness. It was as though she had transformed into a different person. Jane started talking, enjoying meals, and engaging with her family members. Eventually, we were able to discharge her from hospice, as her condition had improved significantly.

Patients may "graduate" from hospice for various reasons. In some cases, their symptoms become manageable, and they are no longer on a rapid decline. The experience is unique for each person, and not everyone will have the opportunity to graduate from hospice care. The key is to enter hospice with an open understanding of the process, ensuring that your loved one receives the best care they deserve.

If your loved one shows improvement, and you feel comfortable considering alternative treatment options or even discontinuing hospice care, you have the flexibility to do so. Ultimately, it is their choice. If they are unable to make decisions for themselves, their designated power of attorney for healthcare can make choices on their behalf.

However, I have also observed cases where families chose to remove a loved one from hospice care for their own reasons, only to later hear that the patient experienced an uncomfortable and distressing death. It is difficult to comprehend why someone would make that decision for their loved one, and I hope this has not been your experience.

One crucial aspect I emphasize is the importance of honoring the patient's wishes whenever possible, especially when they are approaching the end of life. If it can be done safely, fulfilling their final wishes can bring them peace and comfort during this challenging time.

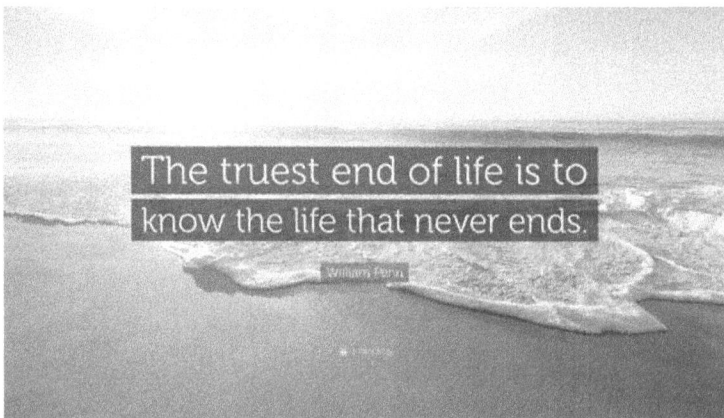

The truest end of life is to know the life that never ends.

William Penn

"I had a friend who worked at a hospice, and he said people in their final moments don't discuss their successes, awards, or what books they wrote or what they accomplished. They only talk about their loves and their regrets, and I think that's very telling."

~ Brad Pitt ~

NOTES

CHAPTER 10

WHAT ABOUT HOSPICE FOR CHILDREN (PEDIATRIC HOSPICE)?

WHAT ABOUT HOSPICE FOR CHILDREN (PEDIATRIC HOSPICE)?

When your loved one is on pediatric hospice, they can continue all treatments for their illness while on hospice. Pediatric hospice care serves as a compassionate and specialized approach to providing comfort, support, and dignity to children facing life-limiting illnesses and their families. This unique form of care recognizes the unique needs of young patients, offering a range of benefits that extend beyond medical treatment alone.

Firstly, pediatric hospice ensures that children can spend their remaining time in a familiar and loving environment—typically their own home. This setting allows them to be surrounded by their family, friends, and cherished possessions, fostering a sense of security and normalcy amidst their challenging circumstances. This environment also promotes bonding and precious moments between the child and their loved ones.

Secondly, pediatric hospice focuses on pain and symptom management, aiming to enhance the child's overall quality of life. A dedicated team of medical professionals, including doctors, nurses, and palliative care specialists, work closely with the family to create a customized care plan that addresses the child's physical, emotional, and psychological needs. This comprehensive approach helps alleviate discomfort and promote a sense of well-being.

Thirdly, pediatric hospice provides invaluable emotional and psychological support for both the child and their family. Social workers, therapists, and counselors play a crucial role in helping families navigate the complex emotions and challenges that come with caring for a seriously ill child. This support extends to siblings, who often require assistance in understanding and coping with their sibling's condition.

Furthermore, pediatric hospice celebrates the uniqueness and individuality of each child. Through art therapy, music therapy, and other creative outlets, children are encouraged to express themselves and leave a legacy. These activities not only provide joyful experiences but also give the family cherished memories to hold onto.

Additionally, pediatric hospice offers respite care to parents and caregivers. The demanding responsibilities of caregiving can take a toll on the family's well-being, and hospice provides intermittent breaks to caregivers, allowing them to rest and recharge. This respite care ensures that caregivers can continue providing their child with the best possible care while also caring for themselves.

In conclusion, pediatric hospice is a profoundly meaningful and essential service that focuses on enhancing the quality of life for children with life-limiting illnesses and their families. By providing holistic care, emotional support, pain management, and opportunities for creative expression, pediatric hospice transforms what might otherwise be a challenging journey into a time of profound connection, comfort, and love.

NOTES

CHAPTER 11

HOW CAN WE PREVENT EXTRA STRESS AT THE END?

HOW CAN WE PREVENT EXTRA STRESS AT THE END?

In cases where a loved one's wishes remain undisclosed, it can lead to family divisions, anger, frustration, and hurtful exchanges among family members. The patient, too, may be affected when they witness these conflicts and disagreements.

I have personally had a will and communicated my wishes for over 30 years. My family is aware of my desires and preferences for the end of life. I strongly recommend taking proactive steps now—regardless of your age or current health status—by completing a living will. By doing so, you can express your wishes to your family, ensuring they are informed about what actions to take if something were to happen to you. This thoughtful preparation can spare your loved ones from the anguish of uncertainty and disagreements during difficult times.

Prevention/Power of Attorney for Health Care and Finances/ Living Will.

I strongly urge you to organize your paperwork well in advance before any crisis arises. I've witnessed numerous family disputes over what they believe their loved one would have wanted at the end of life when there are no written instructions. Each person's preferences can differ significantly—some may desire extensive life-saving measures, while others may prefer a natural conclusion without additional medical interventions like machines, ventilators, or tube feeding.

Preparing these documents is a straightforward process, and you can do it at no cost. Visit your state's official website online, where you can download forms for "power of attorney for health care," "power of attorney for finances," and a "living will." Complete the forms, and then either have them notarized or witnessed by two individuals who are not family members or mentioned in your will. It truly is as simple as that. If you have legal representation, your lawyer may assist you in completing the paperwork.

It's important to note that many people neglect to update these documents after significant life changes, such as divorce or remarriage. I once conducted an educational session in the military regarding this issue, and several attendees had remarried but had not updated their life insurance beneficiaries or power of attorney information, still listing their ex-spouses.

Another unfortunate scenario involved a father who had custody of his children due to the mother's child abuse charges. When the father later fell ill with an incurable disease and passed away, the outdated information meant that the benefits went to his ex-wife instead of his children. Making these changes takes only about 30-40 minutes of your time and can spare your loved ones from arguments and uncertainty during an already challenging time.

Prevention is key whenever possible. The time spent with a loved one and family members at the end of life should be cherished, filled with laughter, love, togetherness, and reminiscing about fond memories—not marred by disputes over their wishes.

"If we listen and observe carefully the dying can teach us important things that we need to learn in preparing for the end of our own life's journey."

~ Robert L. Wise ~

NOTES

CHAPTER 12

WHAT ARE
TOLIET TALKS?

WHAT ARE TOLIET TALKS?

These are significant moments of reflection. It's their way of gradually letting go of their earthly ties and looking ahead to what lies beyond. Please, don't interrupt them during these times. This is their moment, a crucial part of their process as they prepare to bid farewell. They'll reminisce about moments that hold the most significance to them.

As I was wrapping up this book, my mother-in-law received a stage four pancreatic cancer diagnosis. I had the privilege and honor of being by her side during her last few months on this Earth.

It was during those moments when I would assist her to the bathroom that she would become remarkably talkative. She shared stories about each of her children, grandchildren, and great-grandchildren, expressing immense joy and pride in each one of them. She'd also embark on journeys down memory lane, recounting cherished "I remember when" tales, often causing us to burst into fits of laughter. She'd occasionally tease that she needed to use the bathroom more frequently because she was laughing so hard.

Once, while on the toilet, she confided in me about one of her greatest fears: What if she couldn't get up, and none of us girls were around? She would chuckle at the thought. Sadly, her worst fear did become a reality. She couldn't get up when I briefly stepped out for an errand. My husband, her son, kept checking on her, and eventually, she admitted she needed assistance. With a light-hearted comment, he offered, "Mom,

I'll help you up. You can't just sit here until JoAnn gets back." They shared a laugh as he assisted her. She even joked that if it had been her other son, she'd be stuck there all day until I returned to help her up. They laughed again.

It's essential to communicate with your loved one and inquire about their needs. Ask if they have any fears they're grappling with. If they don't feel comfortable discussing it with you, ensure you mention it to the hospice staff during their next visit.

I fondly recall similar moments with my mother while she was under hospice care. We'd sit together and watch Hallmark movies, and she would reminisce about the past. She'd share stories about each of us and the grandchildren. I treasured those precious moments we had together. You learn so much.

The point I wish to emphasize in this chapter is that wherever you find yourself with your loved one, whether they're on the toilet, watching Hallmark movies, or simply resting in bed, listen. They might still have a wealth of stories to share, some of which you may have never heard before.

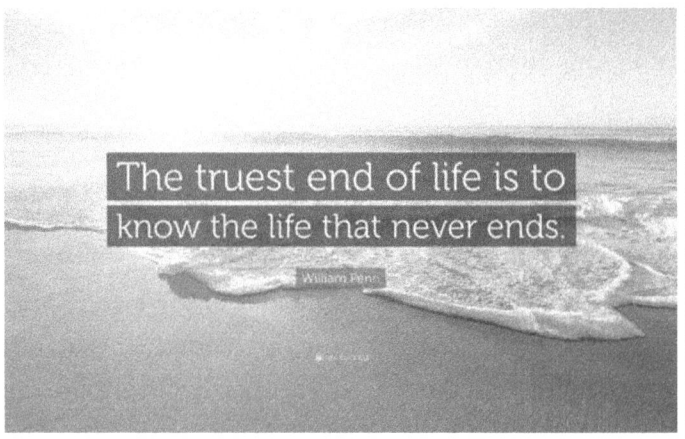

The truest end of life is to know the life that never ends.

William Penn

"I have fought a good fight, I have finished my course, I have kept the faith: Henceforth there is laid up for me a crown of righteousness, which the Lord, the righteous judge, shall give me at that day: and not to me only, but unto all of them also that love his appearing."

~ 2 Timothy 4:7-8 ~

NOTES

CHAPTER 13

Final Thoughts

FINAL THOUGHTS

We've covered an extensive amount of information in this book, and I acknowledge that reading through it may have stirred up a lot of emotions for many of you. I commend you for dedicating your time to empower yourself in handling hospice situations, whether it's for your own future or that of a loved one. Dealing with hospice is undoubtedly challenging, and I would never underestimate the emotional toll it can take.

Having gone through this process multiple times myself, I can genuinely say that I understand the complexities involved. When you're faced with the grief of losing a loved one, it can be overwhelming, and you may find yourself struggling to make the best decisions.

I've witnessed numerous families navigate this difficult journey, and recently, I accompanied a dear friend during their hospice experience. Regrettably, not all families respond optimally to these circumstances, and sometimes, inaction can lead to unfavorable outcomes.

I don't want that to be your experience. While it's undeniably tough, being proactive during this process can help you reach the end with fewer regrets. You've read some of the stories I've shared and received guidance on questions to ask and how to evaluate hospice companies. Now, it's your turn to advocate for your loved one and put this knowledge into practice. While I can't promise perfection (we're all human), you'll be in a much better position by utilizing the tools outlined in this book.

This book is intended to empower you to navigate this process with support. Remember, you're not alone; there are many others facing similar situations. I strongly recommend joining a support group to help you through this journey. The more support, the better.

Don't get me wrong; I've had my own struggles throughout this process. As an example, there was one day when I found myself succumbing to the convenience of fast food and ended up eating it three times in a row. As a nutrition and fitness instructor, I felt disappointed in myself for not practicing what I preach. However, I recognized my missteps and used the experience as a reminder to prioritize healthier choices in the future.

On another occasion, I found myself in the drive-thru lane, about to pay for my meal, when I was informed that the lady in front of me had paid for it. I burst into tears, overwhelmed by the unexpected act of kindness. It was a true blessing and a reassurance that everything would be okay. I was deeply moved by this gesture of generosity during a challenging time.

I was often the only medical professional in the family, and at times, I felt the need to be strong for everyone since I was the hospice nurse. There were instances when I may have been more of a nurse than a daughter or sister, but it's a common response when dealing with such stress. If you ever find yourself in a similar situation, remember to cut yourself some slack and strive to be the person your loved one needs.

Don't hesitate to ask for assistance and communicate your needs with the hospice company. Ask them how to make things happen. Let them serve as your resource guide on this ongoing journey, as that is precisely their role. Hospice will continue to support you for at least a year afterward, which you will undoubtedly need. Various challenges may arise, and you might second-guess your decisions after it's all over. But I want to emphasize: Don't doubt yourself!

During the stressful moments in our lives, we do the best we can. None of us are perfect, but having this knowledge puts you in a better position than those who don't have it.

I receive calls regularly from people seeking help with this process, asking where to turn, how to approach their doctor, and many other legitimate questions. In fact, as I write this final chapter, I am advocating for my uncle to receive hospice care. His primary care physician initially said he didn't qualify and didn't need it. However, after contacting his cardiologist and providing them with relevant information, they realized the necessity and promptly provided the order for hospice care. Sometimes, doctors may not fully understand the situation, and it's crucial to do what's best for your loved one.

Remember the "I remember when" process I introduced earlier? Keep using it throughout the journey, even when you're not in the presence of your loved one. It has the power to bring both laughter and tears to a difficult situation. Trust me, they are aware of how stressful this is for you, and they never wanted you to bear that burden. If they could take it all away from you, they would.

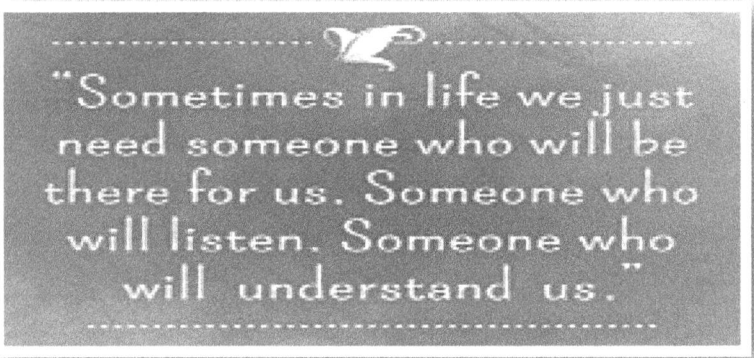

~YOU~

Throughout this challenging process, please remember to prioritize self-care. It's common to see many family members becoming physically and emotionally drained, but that's not the goal. The goal is to attend to what needs to be done and then allow hospice to support you as a valuable resource. Some caregivers may simply need a nap but hesitate to take one, feeling as though they don't have the right to rest. I want to emphasize that you do have that right.

Finally, it's essential to understand that most loved ones prefer not to pass away in your presence. If you happen to leave the room briefly, you may return to find that they've taken their last breath. It's not uncommon for them to choose this moment when you're not there. This happens more frequently than you might realize. I've had the privilege of being the last person some individuals saw before they departed from this world.

HOSPICE STORIES

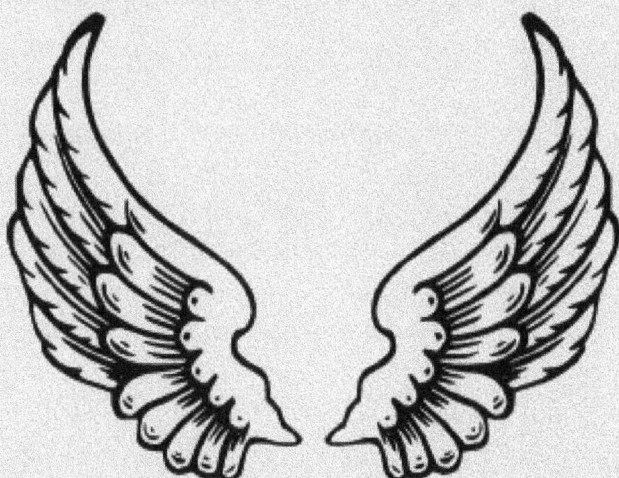

FROM
ME AND MY FRIENDS

~MY BROTHER OTIS'S STORY~

I vividly recall the moment my brother contacted me, describing the little red spots covering his legs. Instinctively, I urged him to go to the emergency room. Following his visit, he received a devastating diagnosis of leukemia in January 2012. During the first month of his hospitalization, we engaged in several conversations about end-of-life scenarios, and I made it clear that I was ready to support him through whatever he needed. I must commend the staff at Methodist Hospital in Omaha, Nebraska, for their excellent care and appreciate their dedication as a nurse myself.

Over the subsequent months, my brother underwent various treatments, but none seemed to be truly effective. In July, he was placed on a trial drug that took a toll on his already weakened system, resulting in multiple hospital admissions due to plummeting blood counts.

I accompanied him to numerous doctor's appointments, and during one of these visits, I inquired about the right time to consider hospice care. The doctor responded, insisting that hospice was not even remotely relevant at that point. She believed he had just embarked on a life-changing treatment and dismissed the idea of hospice care entirely.

While I tend to be an optimist, I also pay attention to the broader context. I didn't want my brother to miss out on precious quality time with his four children. Unfortunately, I witnessed his rapid decline over the next four months, marked by frequent hospital admissions for transfusions and antibiotics.

I distinctly remember a moment in early December when I couldn't accompany him to a doctor's appointment. He had to find an alternate means of transportation and later called me, announcing that he had been admitted to the hospital. That day felt different to me, and I promptly left an important meeting, feeling a deep sense of urgency.

To make a long story short, I remained with my brother during his hospitalization over the next several days. He expressed a desire to see his children, and that day, they all visited him. He appeared remarkably alert and seemed to be having a great day. However, I couldn't shake the feeling that this was the calm before the storm, a moment I had observed in many hospice patients before they experienced a decline.

That night, he began to deteriorate rapidly. I stayed by his side as he went through this difficult process. He had moments of humor, instructing me to prepare the truck for the journey home or asking me to call my husband for a quick departure. At other times, he would wake up and call my name, expressing concern about the impending crowd in his room and urging me to leave if it became too crowded. During this period, a nurse remained with him 24 hours a day due to his worsening condition and the need for constant monitoring.

As a loved one approaches the end of their life, they undergo a profound transition, grappling with the quest to navigate into their next journey. This may manifest as a desire to rise from bed, the sudden impulse to depart from a place, or even moments of agitation, as they contend with uncertainty about their imminent path.

The following day brought more uncertainty, and as night fell once again, his condition deteriorated further. At 2 a.m., three doctors, two nurses, and the crash cart team rushed into his room. I decided it was time to stop the interventions and, eventually, I told the doctor to complete the antibiotics and the blood transfusions after they got him stable.

Throughout his hospital stay, my brother had repeatedly asked me not to let him die in the hospital, and I had promised to do my utmost to honor that request. I called hospice first thing in the morning, explaining the situation. I also asked the doctor, who had been in his room at 2 a.m., to write an order for hospice care, which he agreed to without hesitation.

When the cancer doctor visited my brother's room with four medical students, I confronted her. I informed her that her role in his care was finished, recounting our prior conversation about when it would be time for hospice care and how she had dismissed the idea. I asserted that I was now taking charge of the situation and that she was the one responsible for my brother's deteriorating condition. She protested that I couldn't fire her, to which I reminded her of my authority as his medical power of attorney.

In response, she argued that he wouldn't survive the ambulance ride home. I pointed out that this contradicted her previous insistence on trying another trial drug. I made it clear that my brother's wishes took precedence, and I would not let her or anyone else deny him the opportunity to die at home. We brought my brother home that day, and he spent his final five days on hospice care, celebrating an early Christmas with his children.

I share this story to emphasize the importance of standing up for what you believe is right. Trust your instincts and listen to your loved one's wishes. Be their advocate and honor their desires, even if you're not a medical professional. Pay attention to the bigger picture and remain steadfast in advocating for your loved one's wishes.

~RON LLEWELLYN'S STORY~

One morning, a strong intuition urged me to call my friend Susie, Ron's wife, and advise her to get Ron out of the hospital immediately. Ron had been battling stage four melanoma cancer for a decade, always putting up a resilient fight with periods of remission. This time, he was grappling with excruciating pain, and the medical team had admitted him to the hospital to manage his pain. Unfortunately, after five days in the hospital, his agony showed no signs of abating.

The previous day, the doctors had called Susie to deliver the grim news that Ron's cancer had metastasized extensively, and there were no further treatment options available. Nonetheless, they intended to keep him hospitalized to alleviate his pain. After my conversation with Susie, I firmly believed she needed to take immediate action to fulfill Ron's desire to spend his remaining days at home, surrounded by his family.

While I wasn't entirely certain whether Ron was on the brink of passing away, I had an overwhelming conviction that he should be in the comfort of his home with his loved ones—a calling I attribute to divine wisdom and guidance.

The doctors had refrained from disclosing the full extent of Ron's condition to him, fearing that the news might lead to a decline in his mental and emotional state. I challenged Susie to consider whose life this was—Ron's or the doctors'. I encouraged her to march into the hospital with confidence, assert her authority, and communicate her decision to bring Ron home. (This was during covid.)

I also urged her to have the doctor either visit Ron's hospital room or hold a video call to provide a comprehensive update on his cancer and its spreading. I emphasized that she should not accept any resistance and, should she encounter opposition, to reach out to me for guidance on what to say. I reminded her that both Ron and she had the right to determine his care and choose to bring him home, where he wanted to be.

Susie demonstrated remarkable courage when she confronted the hospital staff. Despite facing resistance, she persisted in advocating for what she knew was best for her husband: bringing him home. That very day, she succeeded in getting Ron discharged from the hospital, and hospice care was initiated the following day.

Ron passed away approximately 30 days later, surrounded by his family. They cherished many precious moments together, filled with laughter, tears, hugs, and heartfelt final exchanges. Ron's wish to die at home, with his family by his side, was granted.

Regrettably, Ron, Susie, and their family had an unfortunate experience with the hospice care they received. Grace, their daughter and a nurse practitioner, contacted me repeatedly, seeking guidance. I explained that this was not how hospice should operate, emphasizing that it should adapt to cater to Ron and his family's unique needs.

The hospice team attempted to dictate their approach without considering Ron and his family's preferences. They were told that certain medications I recommended for pain management were unavailable, but I contacted the pharmacy they used and confirmed that the medications could indeed be obtained.

As the situation deteriorated, Grace, the daughter, had to assume the role of a professional nurse practitioner instead of merely being Ron's daughter. We spent considerable time discussing medications for her father and what she needed to request from the hospice team. Ultimately, there was no room for negotiation; we had to tell them what was needed.

I reached out to the hospice company on several occasions and discovered that their medical director lacked experience in hospice or palliative care. I firmly communicated to the director that Ron's daughter and I would be dictating the care he received.

The chosen hospice company remained unresponsive to the family's wishes, employing a one-size-fits-all approach that did not align with Ron's needs. They misled Ron and his family, failing to provide the care they deserved.

(At this juncture, it's crucial to note that you have the right to change hospice companies.)

During our discussion about that pivotal morning when I called Susie after Ron had passed away, she expressed deep gratitude for my guidance. She believed that if I hadn't intervened, Ron would have passed away in the hospital, alone. This was during the peak of COVID-19 restrictions in hospitals, which meant that she was even denied the opportunity to be by her husband's side. She could only drop off his clothes and nothing more.

Despite the family's negative experience with the hospice company, Ron's wish was granted due to their willingness to speak up and demand the best possible care for him. They respected Ron's desire to spend his final days at home, surrounded by loved ones. In his own home, he received the love and support he needed, and his family had an additional 31 days to share stories, laughter, and tears with him in his final days.

~LORI WOOSLEY-
UDEN'S STORY~

My mom's sugar spiked at the nursing home which landed her in the hospital. Dad stayed with her whilst there, never leaving her side. I arrived and had a serious talk with the nurse to learn this was her end. After all of this sunk in, I called JoAnn, my precious, dear friend who is a hospice nurse.

At the time she was mobilized for the Army and not easy to reach by phone, but God knew I needed her wisdom. When she picked up to hear my update, she told me she could still hear even though she was comatose. She suggested getting people on the phone and putting them on the speaker so they could say their thanksgivings to her, share funny memories and say their farewells.

She shared how I could also talk to her too. I was able to thank her for adopting me, loving me, shaping me into the woman and mom I became. I apologized for when I was a jerk as a teenager, laughed at fun memories we'd made growing up and reminded her how beautiful she was.

We got her grandsons on the phone and her nephews and nieces. Listening to all of this and being by her side, seeing her reactions to their voices was precious and priceless. I got to hold her hand, give her snuggles, give her a damp cloth for her dry mouth and rub her hair.

I put on her favorite songs, prayed with her, and sang hymns. When the nurse came in to talk about hospice, dad asked if we could take her home and found out we could.

I immediately called JoAnn who made phone calls for me and got the wheels moving for this process. Within two hours my mommy was home, in her own bed, just where she'd wanted to be ever since she was admitted into the nursing home.

She spent three months there and now she has got her final wish. Hospice took care of everything. They brought her home, laid her in the bed she'd shared with my dad for over 50 years and taught me how to make her comfortable with pain medications, which I administered throughout the night.

By morning time, I had feelings of regret, like mom would be mad at me for putting this medicine in her mouth. I called JoAnn again, this was the third time, once each day, that when I called, God had her available. She assured me that dying was painful and that I was the one easing that pain for her. JoAnn comforted me as she shared what could happen next and that sometimes our loved ones will take their last breath when we are not there.

I am forever grateful for this knowledge because when I went back to the room where mom was, with dad lying next to her holding her hand, she had already taken her last breath. I am thankful I was prepared so I didn't have to regret leaving her side. I am thankful dad got to spend those last moments with his sweetie. I am thankful beyond words for JoAnn. My mom's passing to eternal life with Jesus was more precious because of my friend and her guidance. Thank you. I love you!

~KELLY W. STORY~

Both of my in-laws were on hospice who died within two months of each other. I spent a huge amount of time with both, so I think I have a pretty good insight into both experiences.

June, my mother-in-law was in hospital hospice at Lakeside. The nurses were fabulous and tried their best to keep her comfortable. The problem was with some of the doctors. It was January and super cold the day the doctors wanted to transfer her to Josie Harper Hospice House. We all knew she was only going to be with us a few days and didn't want her to go through a move, especially in the frigid weather.

I was able to be at the hospital early to catch the doctors on the day of the move and insist she stay. Instead, I ended up blubbering like an idiot and begging. At least it worked and she stayed at the Lakeside hospital. We weren't aware they offered in hospital hospice. We didn't need that stress at that time.

Walt, my father-in-law had all kinds of health problems that got worse after June died. He went to Josie Harper Hospice House. While he was only there for a few days, it couldn't have been a better experience. The whole place made you feel peaceful. The staff went out of their way to make sure not only Walt, but also all of us, were comfortable. It just felt soft if that makes any sense. A soft place to land for the family and a soft place for Walt to die. He passed in the middle of the night in his sleep. The next day they had a candle burning in the entrance. I guess they do this when anyone dies. It was a much better experience than Junes was.

~TRACY HOEFT STORY~

My Dad resided in Memory Care at the Veterans Home in Grand Island. He had recently experienced an episode of aspiration pneumonia, which marked the second occurrence in about three months. Following his improvement, his case manager at the Veterans Home recommended considering Hospice care. Consequently, we arranged a meeting with Hospice, during which they provided a thorough explanation of what Hospice entailed, despite my preexisting knowledge of the concept.

This occurred in April 2010. The nurses were exceptional, and the volunteer assigned to him was truly remarkable. She displayed immense care and affection, reading to him and treating him as if he were her own father. The Hospice team remained attentive and emphasized that being on Hospice care did not equate to receiving no care. For instance, a few weeks before his passing, when his temperature spiked, we were presented with the choice of having blood drawn and initiating antibiotic treatment, a choice we declined in favor of keeping him comfortable.

Recertification to maintain his eligibility for Hospice care occurred multiple times, as his condition improved somewhat in the initial months but not to the extent of discontinuing the service.

When he reached a significant decline in late February 2012, the social worker and nurse accompanied us in making crucial decisions. Members of his Hospice team attended his memorial service, and they continued to provide support in the following weeks. Their follow-ups included inquiring about my mother's well-being. Throughout the first year, they periodically reached out and commemorated his death anniversary with a card for each of us. I am profoundly grateful that we made this choice for him and for ourselves.

On a related note, as palliative care has gained prominence, it is essential for people to grasp the distinction between palliative care and Hospice. Many individuals still associate Hospice primarily with end-stage cancer rather than recognizing its applicability to various end-stage conditions. In my dad's case, he had Alzheimer's.

NOTES

www.ingramcontent.com/pod-product-compliance
Lightning Source LLC
Chambersburg PA
CBHW051247020426
42333CB00025B/3094